1

DEVOTIONAL/ HANDBOOK
FOR
PREGNANT & NURSING
MOTHERS

Dr. Ufuoma Nwachukwu-Onwuka

DR.(MRS). UFUOMA NWACHUKWU-ONWUKA
Email: ufuojaemo@yahoo.com
Tel: +2348036139394, +2348056815965

Contents

DEDICATION

This book is dedicated to mothers all over the world

ACKNOWLEDGEMENT

I give all the glory to God almighty who gave me the inspiration for this book. I wish to appreciate my ever supportive husband for his encouragement. Special thanks to all my children , who God used to give me the "experience" of motherhood. They are all unique. I specially thank my first daughter, Divine, who has given me the push to publish this work which I started writing over five years ago. I abandoned the work, but her coming up with two books at 10, challenged me to finish up. I can not forget to appreciate my mother, Mrs. Janet Ojaemo, who is still mothering me. She is a complete woman, so committed to giving her children the best. She is committed to praying for her children. Some of the concepts in this book, especially in the area of prayers, are what I learnt from her. God has blessed me with wonderful spiritual mothers and great women of faith; Professor(Mrs). Chika Onwasigwe, Barr. Mrs. Joy Ogbonnaya, Rev. Mrs. Nnena Godson, Rev.Mrs. Gloria Ehinloju,Pst. Mrs. Chika Tobi. All these wonderful women, despite their very tight schedule made out time to read and comment on this book, within few days. I am so grateful. Special thanks also to Mrs. Chima Rebacca for editing this book.

FOREWORD

By **Barr. Joy Ogbonnaya and Prof. Chika N. Onwasigwe**

Going through pregnancy could be very challenging for many women. Nursing a baby, especially for first time moms, is no easy feat. Its all about bringing a new life to existence, and so, the author of life Himself cannot be kept aside in this process. I can personally attest that it takes God and knowledge of the basics to successfully go through this phase. 1 can recall my experience during the pregnancies of my three children . Each had its peculiar challenge . The whole experience was full of discomfort ,distress and pain as 1 was barely healthy throughout the 9months. I wake up every day looking at the calendar and counting the days ,meanwhile the journey seemed to be longer. The 9months looked to me like 9years. But the joy of the whole "not too pleasant experience" is the fact that it all ended in praise. 1 put to bed today, and am heading home same day, healthy to begin my normal life.

Dr. Ufuoma Onwuka is my daughter in the Lord. I met her for the first time in 2016, when she invited me as guest minister in her annual Valentine youth conference (True Love Conference) . Since then, we have been relating very well. She is married to a minister of the gospel and she is a speaker in youths, single ladies and women gathering with a burden to reach them ,especially with the message of chastity, making right choices in relationships and having blissful marriages. By God's grace, she has four children.

In this devotional/ hand book, she presents necessary spiritual support and some medical/social tips needed to successfully go through pregnancy and nursing a baby. Also included are scriptural guidelines on raising godly children.

These are practical principles/ guidelines that if followed, pregnancy and nursing a baby will be a successful phase of life. I highly recommend this book to every single and married lady, and men who have women of child bearing age in their lives. This Devotional/

Handbook for pregnant/ nursing mothers is a necessity for newly weds.

Motherhood is a price and it is a priceless gift. If God has made you one, he gives you the capacity to make full proof of it. Read this book and get more determined to fulfill the ministry of motherhood.

Barr. Joy Ogbonnaya
International President, Pleasant Gathering.

***

The beautifully written *Devotional/Handbook for Pregnant/Nursing Mothers* is a treasure and guide for women in their God-given function of reproduction and childrearing. It is a holistic document that dwells on both the spiritual and physical aspects of the mothers in their various situations. Appropriate scriptural passages have been chosen to support each condition ranging from early pregnancy to the nursing of the baby, as well as enhancement of the marriage and the home. Such spiritual advice would greatly benefit all women whose hope is in the victory of Jesus Christ over the schemes of the devil. Health and physical wellbeing advice has equally been given on diverse issues such as adequate nutrition, antenatal care, postnatal care and nurture of the baby. This book should be an invaluable possession in every home and is therefore highly recommended.

Chika N. Onwasigwe
Professor of Community Medicine, College of Medicine, University of Nigeria

COMMENTS

Conception is indeed absolutely of God as the scripture says in Ps.127:3, "Lo children are an heritage of the Lord: and the fruit of the womb is His reward". It is very crucial for us to also know that "it is not of him that willeth nor of him that runneth but of God that showeth mercy" - Rom.9:16. Therefore, I strongly recommend and appreciate this beautiful handbook / devotional for Pregnant and Nursing Mothers.

Rev. Mrs Nnenna Godson - Vice President, Christian Women Fellowship Int'l.

The daily strength that can be drawn from this inspired piece is unparallel. Dr ufuoma has given herself to be used of the Holy Spirit. I read the book, it's a highly recommended daily companion for every pregnant woman and every nursing mother alike. Congratulations to you Dr Ufuoma for this timely piece.

Pst. Mrs Gloria Ehinloju Olubodun

The author of this handbook is a joyful minister of God's WORD, healthcare provider and as a mother of four wonderful children. She undoubtedly has encountered several experiences trying to get pregnant, being pregnant, laboring through childbirth and raising up children and has shared some in this devotional. This book, which I had the privilege of reading, outline some of the challenges would-be mothers and mothers goes through, their causes and biblical approach to these situations with accompanying prayer points to be used to help overcome such challenges. It also contains some medical guidelines on issues relating to pregnancy and nursing a baby.

This is a great treasure to have and it comes handy as a precious marriage gift item for couples. Read this book with the understanding and joy of knowing that you are a partner with God in His plan of procreation.

Yours in His vineyard,
Pst. Mrs.Tobi,Chika
Associate Pastor, Restoration Empower House,
The Redeemed Christian Church of God-North America,
Little Rock, Arkansas, United States of America.

1

I MISSED MY PERIOD!

If you are legally married, then this is always an expected and exciting news. Congratulations! I would say, God has given you the privilege to partner with him in creation. Thank God because the fruit of the womb is a reward from God. You did not conceive because you know the best time to meet with your husband, for some who know better than you, are still waiting on God for this miracle. Thank God for science, but I still remember how I calculated and tried for over a year to get pregnant for my 3rd baby and it did not work. I believe God just wanted to prove to me that He is the one that gives the grace to conceive. On the 22nd of March 2013, God opened my eyes to see the scripture Ruth 4:13. It was God that enabled Ruth to conceive. Give him the glory. IF YOU ARE NOT LEGALLY MARRIED, GOD STILL HAS A PLAN FOR YOU. HE IS A MERCIFUL GOD, AND GOD OF A SECOND

CHANCE. AS YOU REPENT AND TRUST HIM, HE WILL PERFECT ALL THAT CONCERNS YOU.

BIBLE READING AND MEDITATION
Ruth 4:13- So Boaz took Ruth and she became his wife. When he made love to her, the Lord enabled her to conceive, and she gave birth to a son.

PRAYER FOCUS. You can only receive and benefit from God's promises if you are His child. If you wish to receive Jesus as your Lord and saviour, say this prayer.Father, I thank you for sending your son, Jesus, to die for my sins. Lord Jesus, I receive you today as my Lord and saviour. Father, forgive me all my sins. Cleanse me with the blood of Jesus. Cancel my name from the book of death, and write it in the book of life. Satan, I reject you and your works. In Jesus name. Amen.LORD, I thank you for enabling me to carry a seed. I commit myself and this seed unto your hands. May you see me through this period of pregnancy. May I deliver safely, and may I have a healthy baby, in Jesus Name, Amen.

2

GRACE FOR THE JOURNEY

Over the next 38 weeks, it's going to be both an interesting and somehow stressful adventure. You have a role to play in ensuring that this seed in you will come forth and fulfill God's purpose. It's a journey; depend on God to see you through. Committing yourself and this period of your life unto God is necessary, because the devil is always out to steal, kill and destroy. Some have embarked on this journey, and the devil terminated their lives, in the process. The devil knows that when the seed is born, he/she might be a threat to him. Every day and always during this pregnancy period, depend on God, and ask Him for grace.

BIBLE READING AND MEDITATION
2Corin.12:9; But he said to me, "My grace is sufficient for you, for my power is made perfect in weakness." Therefore I will boast all the more

gladly about my weaknesses, so that Christ's power may rest on me.

PRAYER FOCUS- Lord, I receive your grace for this period of pregnancy.

3

GRACE FOR THE JOURNEY-2.

For a lot of women, pregnancy comes with its challenges. From morning sickness, to issues with appetite, weight gain, e.t.c. Some people cannot just live their normal lives during pregnancy, while some are placed on bed rest for months. However, you can believe God for the best.

Jesus has set us free from the curse of the law. For this reason, it is possible to go through pregnancy strong and healthy. Take hold of that which Christ has done for you on the cross. If you have challenges, remember God's word to you is "my grace is sufficient for you". Depend on Him to see you through. He who allowed you to become pregnant, shall not abandon you.

BIBLE READING AND MEDITATION

Isaiah 43:2- When you pass through the waters, I will be with you; and when you pass through the rivers, they will not sweep over you. When you walk through the fire, you will not be burned; the flames will not set you ablaze.

PRAYER FOCUS: Lord, may this pregnancy end in praise. Strengthen me oh Lord. In Jesus name. Amen.

4

BELIEVE GOD FOR NORMAL DEVELOPMENT

When things go wrong during the developmental stage of a baby, it affects the baby throughout life. Although conditions such as learning disorders, motor disorders, autism, language disorders, downs syndrome are genetic and chromosomal, God is able to perfect His work. Believe God and pray that the development of your baby shall be perfect. It is God's desire that our spirit soul and body are perfect. Some children are born with low intelligence quotient and poor ability to comprehend things. As your baby's brain develops, you can ask God for the very best. A high intelligence quotient, ability to articulate properly and reason soundly. God desires that we be the head and not the tail, above always and never beneath.

BIBLE READING AND MEDITATION

Psalm 139:13-14- For you created my inmost being; you knit me together in my mother's womb. I praise you because I am fearfully and wonderfully made;

your works are wonderful, I know that full well.

PRAYER FOCUS: Father, I thank you for this gift you have given me. May you make this baby come out wonderfully. There shall be no defect or abnormality in the developmental process, from the head to toe, In Jesus name, Amen.

5

PERFECT WORK

Apart from praying for the normal development of specific organs and systems, you can also trust God for specific traits, stature, make up,etc You need to pray for wholeness and perfection in the development of your baby from hair to toe. Nothing is too small to ask God. Ask God for the kind of hair you want your baby to have. I know you would prefer your baby girl not to have scanty hair. Why not you pray about it? What about the height? Do you want a short son or daughter, what about the complexion and the voice? Some people's voices sound like angels. Which do you want? The size of the head, ear, nose, mouth, etc- you can determine all these qualities in the place of prayer. In as much as these features has to do with the genetic make-up of an individual, God, who is the author and finisher is able to perfect all things. When I had my first baby, almost everybody that came around the hospital ward that day were attracted to the baby. She looked wonderful. I actually prayed about those tiny details. Ask and receive, that your joy may be complete (John16:24). God cares about your "tiny details".

BIBLE READING AND MEDITATION
Psalm 138:8 (KJV)

The Lord will perfect that which concerneth me: thy mercy, O Lord, endureth for ever: forsake not the works of thine own hands.

PRAYER FOCUS: Father, perfect every thing that has to do with the development of this baby. May he/she be WONDERFULLY made in Jesus name. Pray about specific areas of concern.

6

DO NOT BE CARELESS

Do not take things for granted during your pregnancy. Keep your medical appointments, report any abnormal signs/feeling to your doctor. Take your routine drugs, and the recommended dozes, take your vaccinations. According to centres for disease control and prevention, you are to seek medical help if there is :pain of any kind, strong cramps, contractions at 20 minute internal, vaginal bleeding or leaking of fluid, dizziness or fainting, shortness of breath, heart palpitation, constant nausea and vomiting, trouble walking, oedema(swelling of joints),decreased activity of baby. As you pray, do not be careless about WATCHING!

BIBLE READING AND MEDITATION
Ephesians 6:18 New International Version (NIV)

18 And pray in the Spirit on all occasions with all kinds of prayers and requests. With this in mind,

be alert and always keep on praying for all the Lord's people.

PRAYER FOCUS: Father, as I do all that is expected of me during this pregnancy, may you crown my efforts with great testimony in Jesus name, Amen.

7

NO LOSS, NO DEATH

In God's plan, it takes an average of 9 months for a baby to get mature in the womb before being brought into the world. Though premature babies could survive, it is better to have the best. Trust God today that you will not have a premature baby.

God's will for you is that your vine shall not cast her fruit before the time(Malachi 3:11). Believe and receive His promise. Believe God that you shall not miscarry. Also have faith in God that according to His word He shall save you in childbearing.(I Timothy 2:15)You shall not die.

His will is that He who caused you to be pregnant will bring you to the end, which is delivery. It is the enemy that steals, kills and destroys. But let not your heart be troubled. Jesus can give life and life in abundance. Daily cover your baby with the blood of Jesus. He who started a good work will see it to completion.

BIBLE READING AND MEDITATION

Phil. 1:6-Being confident of this, that he who began a good work in you will carry it on to completion until the day of Christ Jesus.

Exodus 23:26(NIV)- And non will miscarry or be barren in your land. I will give you a full life span.

PRAYER FOCUS: Appreciate God for another day. Father, watch over this pregnancy. According to your word, I shall not miscarry. I shall not have still birth. The pregnancy shall be full-term, and I shall deliver a healthy baby, in Jesus name, Amen.

8

THE WHOLE ARMOUR

Bearing in mind that the devil targets the children of God to try to make God's word less effective in their lives, you cannot help but be strong in faith. You must make deliberate efforts to put on the whole armour of God, so that the enemy would have no ground/power against you. Make out time to still study or listen to God's word. In fact, literally force yourself to eat the word, just like someone who is ill forces himself to take physical food even when there is no appetite, so he can get well faster. Be strong in the lord and in the power of his might. Put on the shield of faith. When the devil brings negative thoughts of how the baby could die during delivery, resist him with God's word in faith.

BIBLE READING AND MEDITATION
Ephesians 6:11-12 (KJV)

Put on the whole armour of God, that ye may be able to stand against the wiles of the devil. For we wrestle not against flesh and blood, but against principalities, against powers, against the rulers of the darkness of this world, against spiritual wickedness in high places.

PRAYER FOCUS: Appreciate God for a new day. Lord, I receive strength to put on my whole armour. Help me to fight the good fight of faith and come out victoriously, in Jesus name, Amen.

9

THE PERSON OF THE HOLY SPIRIT

The period of pregnancy is a season of war as the enemy would do all things possible to ensure that your seed does not live. (Rev 12:1) because he knows that if he allows that seed, it will bruise his heel. Only your relationship with God can grant you victory in this season. You need to stand in the power of the Holy Spirit. The Holy Spirit is sent to help you overcome the wiles of the enemy. Always be sure you are connected to him. Don't allow the devil take away your child while you are sleeping (unconsciousness), as is the case in 1 kings 3: 16-20. Be sensitive, the Holy Spirit will reveal the plans of the enemy and strengthen you to pray.

BIBLE READING AND MEDITATION

Romans 8:26- In the same way, the Spirit helps us in our weakness. We do not know what we ought to pray for, but the Spirit himself intercedes for us through wordless groans.

1Corin.2:10-These are the things God has revealed to us by his Spirit. The Spirit searches all things, even the deep things of God.

PRAYER FOCUS: Appreciate God for a new day. Holy spirit, be my senior partner throughout this journey and always. Help me to follow your leading, in Jesus name, Amen.

EAT THE RIGHT FOOD

The development of your baby to a large extent depends on what you eat. Eat healthy meals. It is necessary to know that what you eat would eventually reflect on the health of the baby. Take more of proteins, vitamins and minerals. Eat folate-rich food like oranges, fortified cereals etc. Avoid gaining too much weight ,which might be difficult to lose later, or make your baby too big and make delivery difficult. According to the guidelines for institute of medicine, based on a woman's body mass index(BMI) before pregnancy,

Under weight should gain 28-40pounds

Normal weight   25-35 pounds

Overweight 15-25 pounds

obese   11-20pounds

BIBLE READING AND MEDITATION

1Corin 10:31- So whether you eat or drink or whatever you do, do it all for the glory of God.

Isaiah 55:2 (NIV)-Why spend money on what is not bread, and your labour on what does not satisfy? Listen, listen to me, and eat what is good, and you will delight in the richest of fare.

PRAYER FOCUS: Appreciate God for a new day. Father, as I take the right decision concerning what I eat, may such be for the health and nourishment of the baby and me, in Jesus name. Amen.

11

THINGS TO AVOID

Smoking

Apart from pregnancy, note that smoking is generally dangerous to your health. Exposure to second hand smoke is as dangerous as partaking in it. Do not destroy God's temple. According to studies, women who smoke during pregnancy are likely to have children who have learning disabilities. Such children are also more likely to try smoking at an earlier age and become regular smokers earlier due to physiologic nicotine addiction (Kimberly Holland,2019). Second hand smoke is dangerous to your baby.

BIBLE READING AND MEDITATION

1 Corin3:16-17-Do you not know that you are God's temple and that God's Spirit dwells in you? If anyone destroys God's temple, God will destroy him. For God's temple is holy, and you are that temple.

PRAYER FOCUS: Appreciate God for a new day. Oh lord, as I consciously avoid everything that could be harmful to me and my baby, crown my efforts with testimony. In Jesus name. Amen.

12

THINGS TO AVOID 2

Alcohol

Alcohol is generally dangerous to your health, but in pregnancy, it could lead to having a baby with complications. It can also cause premature delivery, congenital disabilities and under weight(American Academy of Pediatrics). They advice, that no amount of alcohol intake is considered safe during pregnancy, and there is no safe trimester to drink alcohol.

Avoid caffeine (tea and coffee, cola and other soft drink that contain caffeine. They are linked to miscarriage and low birth weight(American Journal of Obstetrics and Gynecology).

Moreover, avoid heavy lifting, standing for a long period , eating raw /uncooked meat and eggs, unpasteurized cheese as these lead to infection with toxoplasmosis or salmonella.Also wash hands thoroughly after handling raw meat. Avoid liver and other foods, rich in vitamin A.

Avoid very hot environment,saunas. Avoid fishes that contain mercury.

BIBLE READING AND MEDITATION

Prov 23;31-32-Do not gaze at wine when it is red, when it sparkles in the cup,
when it goes down smoothly! In the end it bites like a snake   and poisons like a viper.
1Corin. 6:12(KJV)-All things are lawful unto me,but all things are not expedient:all things are lawful for me, but i will not be brought under the power of any.

PRAYER FOCUS: Appreciate God for a new day. Oh lord, as I consciously avoid everything that could be harmful to me and my baby, crown my efforts with testimony. In Jesus name. Amen.

13

ORDAINED FROM THE WOMB

God makes no mistake. Before each child is formed in the womb, God has a definite plan for that child. The one you are carrying is not different. The unfortunate thing is that many end up not fulfilling that plan. The parents of Samson had a role to play in helping their son to fulfill his purpose and destiny. They were to ensure that no razor touches his hair, that he takes no fermented drink and eat nothing unclean(Judges 13:3-9). Mother you too have a role to play in ensuring that your baby fulfills God's plan. To begin with, you need to pray according to 1 Tim 1:18. There is a war the enemy is launching to ensure the plan of God is not fulfilled. You must fight the good fight of faith, with the prophecy that has gone ahead. The battle starts from the womb. Pray, mothers, pray!

BIBLE READING AND MEDITATION

Jer. 1 : 5-Before I formed you in the womb I knew you,before you were born I set you apart;I appointed you as a prophet to the nations."

PRAYER FOCUS: Appreciate God for a new day. Lord, I dedicate this baby in my womb to you. The devil cannot stop him/ her. He/she shall fulfill purpose and destiny. In Jesus name. Amen.

14

PREPARING FOR DELIVERY

Note that your delivery could come either two weeks before or after your expected date of delivery(EDD). It is expected that you get all your delivery items ready in a bag. Your husband, or someone you expect to be available at the appointed time should be aware of the location of the bag. Having a baby is not an emergency; it takes nine months, and so, it is not wise to be unprepared. Funny enough, some women approach their due date without adequate preparation. I was once in the labour room, when one lady was brought in for delivery. She said she went to the market to shop for delivery items, when she began to have labour pains. What if her labour started the night prior to that? She would have been stranded. You do not have to wait till your third trimester to start buying your needed items. You may be overwhelmed and it would look like a big project.You can buy them gradually, even from the first trimester. Most hospitals have their list of required items. Get the list early enough, and start preparing.

BIBLE READING AND MEDITATION
Prov 6:6-8 (NIV)-Go to the ant, you sluggard;consider its ways and be wise!It has no commander,no overseer or ruler,yet it stores its provisions in summer and gathers its food at harvest.

PRAYER FOCUS: Appreciate God for a new day. Lord, I choose to be wise and prepare ahead, like the ant. Supply all my needs oh God. In Jesus name. Amen.

15

PREPARING FOR DELIVERY-2

The most important aspect of preparation for delivery, is the need to prepare your heart. You may have heard lots of negative stories about labour and delivery, but you can choose what to believe. Also remember, that you get what you believe. Faith attracts positive things, while fear attracts the negative. The truth still remains that there are people who do not have labour pains or experience prolonged labour; you can believe God for the best. But whether painful or not, trust God to have a safe delivery, with baby and mother alive and healthy. All through your pregnancy, get to know God's promises about delivery. Study the scriptures and have them in your heart. Be positive about labour and delivery.

BIBLE READING AND MEDITATION
Psalm 55:22 "Cast all your anxiety on him because **he cares for you.**" (ESV)

Isaiah 41:10 "Do not fear, for I am with you; do not be dismayed, for I am your God. **I will strengthen you and help you**; I will uphold you with my righteous right hand." (NIV)

2 Timothy 4:17 "But the Lord stood by me and **strengthened me**." (ESV)

Psalm 46:1-3 "**God is our refuge and strength**, a very present help in trouble. Therefore we will not fear though the earth gives way, though the mountains be moved into the heart of the sea, though its waters roar and foam, though the mountains tremble at its swelling." (ESV)

Prov.31:25- Strength and honour are her clothing:and she shall rejoice in time to come.

Exo. 1;19 (NIV)-The midwives answered Pharaoh, "Hebrew women are not like Egyptian women; they are vigorous and give birth before the midwives arrive."

Psalm 56:3 "When I am afraid, **I put my trust in you**." (NIV)

Isaiah 66:9(NIV)-Do I bring to the moment of birth and not give delivery?" says the Lord. "Do I close up the womb when I bring to delivery?" says your God.

PRAYER FOCUS: Appreciate God for a new day. Lord, I appreciate you because you are not a man that you should lie. You will fulfil your promises to me. I refuse to fear. I shall deliver safely, in Jesus name. Amen.

16

IN THE FAVOUR ROOM

God's word says, when Zion travailed, he brought forth(Isaiah 66:8). Believe God that you shall bring forth. Take over the atmosphere of the labour ward for God. Invite His presence. Release angels, cover yourself, your baby, the atmosphere and the attendants with the blood of Jesus. Ask God to use them to help you, directing their actions and decisions. Some persons have lost their lives and/or their baby due to carelessness of medical staff. Pray that they shall not make mistakes.

BIBLE READING AND MEDITATION
1 Tim. 2:15(NIV) But women will be saved through childbearing—if they continue in faith, love and holiness with propriety.

Rev. 12:1-6-And there appeared a great wonder in heaven; a woman clothed with the sun, and the moon under her feet, and upon her head a crown of twelve stars:

2 And she being with child cried, travailing in birth, and pained to be delivered.

3 And there appeared another wonder in heaven; and behold a great red dragon, having seven heads and ten horns, and seven crowns upon his heads.

4 And his tail drew the third part of the stars of heaven, and did cast them to the earth: and the dragon stood before the woman which was ready to be delivered, for to devour her child as soon as it was born.

5 And she brought forth a man child, who was to rule all nations with a rod of iron: and her child was caught up unto God, and to his throne.

6 And the woman fled into the wilderness, where she hath a place prepared of God, that they should feed her there a thousand two hundred and threescore days.

PRAYER FOCUS: Appreciate God for this day. Lord, I worship you. Father, I welcome your presence. Jesus, I welcome your presence. Holy Spirit, come and take over this atmosphere. I rebuke the spirit of fear. Satan I come against your works in Jesus name. Sing worship songs and pray the scriptures all through.

17

YOU SHALL NOT LABOUR IN VAIN

The joy of many who were supposed to be celebrating after delivery, have been truncated many times, due to either the loss of a baby or the mother during or after birth. Some have gone to the hospital with baby things, hoping to come back after few hours with their babies, but the enemy had a plan too. This you must stand against.

When I was in labour for my second child, I could almost audibly hear the devil say that I would not have the baby alive, or that I would die. Though very painful, the contractions/dilation was progressing so fast, that the nurses had brought out my baby's things, including the dress, she would put on after delivery.The devil spoke that she wouldn't wear the dress. There I was for hours, in pains and baby couldn't descend for me to push. I got so exhausted, but I held on to God's word. I continuously spoke out loud, "I shall not die". I quoted what God says about delivery, that He shall save me in child bearing. To God be the glory, He proved the devil a liar. Baby later came out with her face up (occipitoposterior position). My labour was not in vain to God's glory. Both of us are alive to fulfill God's purpose. Mothers, you must stand against the wiles of the devil. You must not be told sorry, but congratulations.

BIBLE READING AND MEDITATION

Isaiah 65:23(NIV)-They will not labour in vain, nor will they bear children doomed to misfortune; for they will be a people blessed by the lord, they and their descendants with them.

Isaiah 66:8 (KJV)

Who hath heard such a thing? who hath seen such things? Shall the earth be made to bring forth in one day? or shall a nation be born at once? for as soon as Zion travailed, she brought forth her children.

PRAYER FOCUS: Appreciate God for this great day. Lord, according to your word, I shall not labour in vain. As I travail, I shall bring forth. I will be healthy and the baby will be healthy too. In Jesus name. Amen.

18

HERE THE BABY COMES

Congratulations dear mother. Once again, it is a privilege for God to have chosen you, as a partner in bringing forth this wonderful being. Never forget that many are still trusting God for this miracle. This should help and make you forget whatever pains/ discomfort you went through during pregnancy, in the labour and delivery rooms. Not all that went in there come out alive. Some did but without their babies. Why not appreciate God for His faithfulness.

BIBLE READING AND MEDITATION
John 16:21(NIV)-A woman giving birth to a child has pain because her time has come; but when her baby is born she forgets the anguish because of her joy that a child is born into the world.
Psalm 113:9 (KJV)
He maketh the barren woman to keep house, and to be a joyful mother of children. Praise ye the Lord.

PRAYER FOCUS: Appreciate God for this great day. Lord, you are great, and there is none like you. Thank you for seeing me through. Thank you Lord for safe delivery. Thank you for giving me joy in the morning. Be praised for ever. In Jesus name. Amen.

19

DEDICATION

As a Christian, we know there is a day of baby dedication in churches. However, as one who has a relationship with God, you need to dedicate your child before birth but practically at birth. This is necessary before the enemy who comes to steal, kill and destroy starts working. Sweet mother I hope you do not see it, as too early to settle the future of your baby in the place of prayer. Commit every aspect of his/her life unto God, that He alone shall be in charge, that the devil will have no place in him/her.

BIBLE READING AND MEDITATION
1 Samuel 1:27-28 (KJV)

27 For this child I prayed; and the Lord hath given me my petition which I asked of him:

28 Therefore also I have lent him to the Lord; as long as he liveth he shall be lent to the Lord. And he worshipped the Lord there.

Luke 2:22-When the time came for the purification rites required by the Law of Moses, Joseph and Mary took him to Jerusalem to present him to the Lord.

PRAYER FOCUS: Appreciate God for a new day. Father, I dedicate this baby to you. Take charge of his/ her life. Frustrate the counsel of the enemy over him/ her. May he/ she fulfil purpose and destiny. In Jesus name. Amen.

20

THE NAME MATTERS

The importance of a name is evident in the fact that, on various occasions, God himself was involved in naming people. The name of a child speaks into the life and destiny of the child. It is actually your prophetic declaration over that child. Whenever you call that child, you are actually invoking the meaning of that name over that child. Have you ever wondered why God changed Abram's name to Abraham, and Sarai's name to Sarah? Their story needed to change. Their name needed to reflect what they were expecting. Abram wanted a child and God changed his name to Abraham which means father of nations. Whenever his family, friends or neighbours called him, Abraham, they were declaring that he was father of nations, even though he did not have a child then. But you know the story, he actually became the father of nations.

BIBLE READING AND MEDITATION

Prov.22:2-A good name is rather to be chosen than great riches, and loving favour rather than silver and gold.

Genesis   2:19

(KJV)

And out of the ground the LORD God formed every beast of the field, and every fowl of the air; and brought them unto Adam to see what he would call them: and whatsoever Adam called every living creature, that was the name thereof.

PRAYER FOCUS: Appreciate God for a new day. Lord, as you lead my husband and me in naming this baby, he/ she shall answer to that name. In Jesus name. Amen.

21

THE NAME MATTERS-2

Still on the issue of naming, let's consider that God changed Jacob's name to Israel. Jacob's life was patterned after his name. He was a supplanter. But when he was in the womb, the Lord told the mother "two NATIONS are in your womb"(Gen. 25:23). But the parents called him a supplanter. In order to fulfill purpose and destiny, God had to change his name, to Israel; a great NATION. Can you also remember Jabez? How his life was full of sorrow because of his name?(1 Chron. 4:9-10) . He had to pray for God to enlarge his coast, before he got a breakthrough.

Parents are encouraged to be careful about the names they give their children. Both parents should agree on this.

BIBLE READING AND MEDITATION

Luke 1:59-63 On the eighth day they came to

circumcise the child, and they were going to name him after his father Zechariah, 60 but his mother spoke up and said, "No! He is to be called John."

61 They said to her, "There is no one among your relatives who has that name."

62 Then they made signs to his father, to find out what he would like to name the child. 63 He asked for a writing tablet, and to everyone's astonishment he wrote, "His name is John."

PRAYER FOCUS: Appreciate God for a new day. Lord, as you lead my husband and me in naming this baby, he/she shall answer to that name. In Jesus name. Amen.

22

BE SENSITIVE

The devil has not changed. Note that the star of your child has appeared and the enemy is not happy. He could come in disguise as a visitor. Be sensitive in spirit as people pay you visit. Some come with evil intension. Note that not all that come around should have access to your baby. That's why you must make out time to be connected to God despite the much attention that the baby demands. If you do not have peace in your mind about a visitor having access to your baby, do not try to please anyone by going against your spirit. If for any reason, anyone has access, and you are not comfortable, pray immediately, and cover your child with the blood of Jesus, cancelling and nullifying whatever the enemy has done.

BIBLE READING AND MEDITATION
Matt. 2: 7-8,13-16.(KJV)

7 The Herod, when he had privily called the wise men, enquired of them diligently what time the star appeared.

8 And sent them to Bethlehem, and said, Go and search diligently for the young child; and when ye have found him, bring me word again, that I may come and worship him also.

13 And when they departed, behold the angel of the Lord appeareth to Joseph in the dream, saying, Arise, and take the young child and his mother, and flee into Egypt, and be thou there until I bring thee word: for Herod will seek the young child to destroy him.

14 When he arose, he took the young child and his mother by night, and departed into Egypt:

15 And was there until the death of Herod: that it might be fulfilled which was spoken of the Lord by the prophet, saying, Out of Egypt have I called my son.

16 Then Herod, when he saw that he was mocked of the wise men, was exceeding wroth, and sent forth, and slew all the children that were in

Bethlehem, and in all the coasts thereof, from two years old and under, according to the time which he had diligently inquired of the wise men.

PRAYER FOCUS: Appreciate God for a new day. Father, help me to be sensitive to your leading over my baby. Frustrate every plan of the enemy. In Jesus name. Amen.

23

I STILL LOVE YOU.

Nursing a baby at the early stage could really be tasking: waking up several times at night to feed the baby, and still not able to sleep properly during the day because you still have to attend to him/her. Worse still if the baby is the type that would not allow anyone else to carry him or her. Sometimes she would even bite your breast while breastfeeding. You could really be worn out sometimes and may feel like beating the little baby. Let the joy of being a mother overwhelm you. Remember too that in all your naughtiness, God never forsook you. Even when you were a sinner, he bore pains for your sake.

BIBLE READING AND MEDITATION
Romans 8:35-37- (KJV)

35 Who shall separate us from the love of Christ? shall tribulation, or distress, or persecution, or famine, or nakedness, or peril, or sword?

36 As it is written, For thy sake we are killed all the day long; we are accounted as sheep for the slaughter.

37 Nay, in all these things we are more than conquerors through him that loved us.

PRAYER FOCUS: Appreciate God for a new day. Lord, thank you for the privilege of being a mother. No matter the pain and inconveniences, help me to continually care for my baby. I receive joy. In Jesus name. Amen

24

I STILL LOVE YOU-2.

I had often wondered at what the scripture says:"even if a mother forgets the suckling child, God will not forget us". But why would a mother forget the suckling child. I wondered. Now I understand – there could be pain associated with child bearing. Just from the delivery room, you could be faced with the pain of an episiotomy, tear or CS, breast feeding could bring pain due to sore nipples, and then, the stress from sleepless night. Sometime the mother wishes the baby would understand that she is in pain and refrain from "stressing her" by asking for more breast milk or crying and seeking for attention, but sorry it can't. Mother, you have to endure the pain and still lovingly attend to the baby, husband etc- trusting that God would reward you. Soon, it will be over, the baby will grow up and "make you proud".

BIBLE READING AND MEDITATION
Hebrews 12:2- (NIV)

Fixing our eyes on Jesus, the pioneer and perfecter of our faith. For the joy set before him he endured the cross, scorning its shame, and sat down at the right hand of the throne of God.

PRAYER FOCUS: Appreciate God for a new day. I receive grace to love and care for my baby today and always, in Jesus name. Amen.

25

MUMMY! MUMMY!! MUMMY!!!

Sometimes, the nursing mother gets engrossed with taking care of the new baby, that she unconsciously, but literarily abandons the other children. They call for mummy's attention, but do not get it. Sometimes, the older child becomes jealous of the little baby, that he/she ends up beating the tiny baby. Dear mum, the older child needs your attention too. Deliberately create time to attend to him/her. Find out why he is calling. Listen to him, touch him/her, reaffirm that you still care, help him or her understand that she has a sibling now, that needs care and more attention, like you gave him/her when he was smaller. Explain, that as a "big" brother / sister, she should also care for the baby.

BIBLE READING AND MEDITATION
Prov.31:27-28

She looks well to the ways of her household and does not eat the bread of idleness. Her children rise up and call her blessed; her husband also, and he praises her.

PRAYER FOCUS: Appreciate God for a new day. Father, despite the demands of caring for a new baby, give me grace to look to the ways of my HOUSEHOLD. May I not neglect anyone. In Jesus name. Amen.

26

WHAT GOD HAS JOINED TOGETHER.

Nursing a baby could keep you so busy and tired that you may want to or there is tendency to forget the vow you made to your husband, to be committed to him always. What God has joined together, let not the baby put asunder. Make out time to still love your husband, allow him to love you. Don't allow the oil of marriage to run dry. Do not give the enemy a chance to operate and distract him. During the period of pregnancy and then shortly after delivery, he might have had to abstain from sex over a long period(note that it is not wrong to have sex during pregnancy except there are indications against it). Do try to make yourself available for sex as soon as possible. Even if you have a tear or stitches, you can still find ways to get him satisfied without penetrations.

BIBLE READING AND MEDITATION

Mark 10:9-What therefore God has joined together, let not man separate

PRAYER FOCUS: Appreciate God for a new day. Lord, help me to fulfil my marital vows even in times like this. Help me to love my husband.

27

GOD SHALL SUPPLY

Considering the current economic situation in most places, raising a child is no small feat. From buying of diapers, to some immunizations you need to pay for, to feeding, especially after exclusive breastfeeding is over, to clothing, it is quite expensive to raise a child. However, you must understand that this is God's project. He shall keep his word.

BIBLE READING AND MEDITATION
Philippians 4:19 (KJV)-But my God shall supply all your need according to his riches in glory by Christ Jesus.

PRAYER FOCUS: Appreciate God for a new day. God, supply everything I need to care for this baby. In Jesus name. Amen.

28

EXCLUSIVE BREASFEEDING; ENCOURAGED

Exclusive breastfeeding has been discovered to be the best for the first 6 months of life. It is meant to be simplest too as it is cost effective (though the mother has to eat very good food). It is less stressful as you do not have to prepare it and wash plate(you only need to keep your body clean and wash your hands). But surprisingly a lot of mothers see it as a burden, especially because, it automatically makes them always have to be with the child. Thank God for technology, breast pumps are now available. You can extract breast milk and preserve for your baby while you are on the go. The benefits of exclusive breastfeeding cannot be over emphasized.

BIBLE READING AND MEDITATION
Galatians 6:9 (KJV)

And let us not be weary in well doing: for in due season we shall reap, if we faint not.

PRAYER FOCUS: Appreciate God for a new day. Father help me to make the sacrifice of exclusive breastfeeding for 6months. Your grace is sufficient for me. Thank you Lord. In Jesus name. Amen.

29

BY HIS WOUNDS WE ARE HEALED

The arrival of a new baby could sometimes be with mixed feelings. Yes happy that a child is born, but unhappy because of pains. I can't forget in a hurry the pains I went through after giving birth to each of my children.

In the case of my first baby, I had an episiotomy. For the other two, I had tear . For my 3rd baby, the suture got broken and I was asked to go for re-suturing. Considering the pain that could be involved, I opted for anti-biotics, although I was told that there is possibility of the wound healing without proper alignment. I heard lots of comments that filled my heart with trepidation, but God gave me his word in Ezekiel 37; that the bones located their bones and the sinews and the flesh came upon them. I held unto that word, and to God's glory, I was perfectly healed without having to go for re-suturing. There was restoration to the former anatomical position.

Child of God, what are you passing through as a health condition, due to your baby's birth process? Is it pregnancy induced diabetes or hypertension? Did you have a Caesarean section? By his wounds you are healed. Receive that which Christ has done for you. Confess it, and it shall come to manifestation.

BIBLE READING AND MEDITATION
Isaiah 53:5 - (NKJV)
But He was wounded for our transgressions. He was bruised for our iniquities;
The chastisement for our peace was upon Him. And by His stripes we are healed.

PRAYER FOCUS: Appreciate God for a new day. God, I receive healing concerning any health challenge I am currently facing as a result of conception and delivery. Thank you Lord, in Jesus name. Amen.

30

NONE OF THESE DISEASES SHALL COME NEAR YOU.

Children are prone to a number of diseases, especially due to their low immunity. Also, they have little control over their environment, and do not practise good hygiene. Some of these diseases are ; Pneumonia, diarrhoea, malaria, measles. According to UNICEF factsheet in 2015, malaria kills 1,200 children every day, and children under the age of 5 represent 78 percent of global malaria deaths. Mothers, let us play our role in ensuring that our children are not exposed to diseases/infections by using mosquito nets, washing hands and utensil properly and also keeping your house neat-to prevent diarrhoea, giving them the necessary vaccinations and going for prompt medical attention when necessary. We must ultimately hold on to God's word for he does not lie. He said -none of these diseases shall come near your dwelling. Your child has heavenly immunity. You do not have to allow fear come into your heart, for fear is a spirit that attracts what you fear, just as faith attracts the good things you expect. God's word says, the child shall not die till he is a 100 years old(Isaiah 65:20).

BIBLE READING AND MEDITATION

Exo. 23:25-And ye shall serve the LORD your God, and he shall bless thy bread, and thy water; and I will take sickness away from the midst of thee.(KJV)

PRAYER FOCUS: Appreciate God for a new day. Father, as I play my role in taking good care of my baby, he/she shall not contract any form of the diseases or infection. He/she shall live in good health all the days of his/her life. In Jesus name. Amen

31

IMMUNIZATION SCHEDULE

Some mothers for one reason or the other, fail to give their children the necessary immunization, either completely, or at the right time. This could have adverse effect on the baby later in life. It is necessary to take note of the various immunization, and the right time for them to be taken, and follow it.

According to WHO, the following is the vaccination schedule at each age.

AT BIRTH: Hepatitis B, Oral Polio(OPV),BCG.

AT 6 WEEKS: Oral Polio(OPV),Hepatitis B, DPT(Diphtheria,Tetanus&Pertusis),Hib(Haemophi lus influenza type b), Rotavirus(diarrhea and vomiting),Pneumococcal conjugate(Pneumonia and Otitis media).

AT 10 WEEKS:Oral Polio(OPV),Hepatitis B, DPT, Hib, Rotavirus,Pneumococcal conjugate.

AT 14 WEEKS:Oral Polio(OPV),Hepatitis B, DPT,Hib ,Pneumococcal conjugate.
AT 9 MONTHS: Measles and Yellow fever.
AT 12-15 MONTHS: MMR(Measles, Mumps & Rubella),Chicken pox,Pneumococcal conjugate.
AT 18 MONTHS: DPT(Booster), OPV(Booster)
FROM 2 YEARS: Typhoid fever, Meningitis.

BIBLE READING AND MEDITATION
Prov.4:7-Wisdom is the principal thing; therefore get wisdom: and with all thy getting get understanding.

PRAYER FOCUS: Appreciate God for a new day. Lord, by your spirit, help me to always remember the due date for my baby's immunizations. I also ask for your provision, to be able to afford those vaccines that I need to pay for. In Jesus name. Amen.

32

THERE SHALL BE NO DELAY

As a child is born, there is a normal developmental process the child should go through. For example, at age one month, your child should be able to close eyes in bright light and open eyes in dim light, should be sensitive to loud noises and mother's voice. At 2 months, a child should be able to lift its head (have neck control). However sometimes you see a child of 2 years that has not walked. That is kind of abnormal. A child at 3years that can not talk is abnormal. That is why you as a mother must start praying even from when your baby is in the womb and continue when he/she is born to ensure that there is no delay in any developmental process.

However, it is also important that the baby is fed with the right meal to ensure proper development. Even if he/she is on exclusive breastfeeding, the mother should feed properly(balanced diet).

BIBLE READING AND MEDITATION
Luke2:40

And the child grew and became strong; he was filled with wisdom ,and the grace of God was on him.

PRAYER FOCUS: Appreciate God for a new day. Father, there shall be no delay. My baby shall achieve each developmental milestone in due season.

33

MILESTONES CONTINUED

Between one to three months, a baby may start to smile initially to him/herself, but later in response to your smile, grip objects in the hand, raise head and chest when lying prostrate. At 3 months, a baby should be able to support itself when held on fore arms, should be able to lift foot while lying, have head eye coordination and eye hand co-ordination, can open hand, can vocalize. At 6 months your baby should be able to sit, turn over unaided, enjoy music/rhythym, etc. At 12 months the child should be able to walk, put cube in a cup, react to strangers, enjoy using common objects as toy, musical toys, respond when name is called. Report any prolonged delay in development early enough.

BIBLE READING AND MEDITATION
Luke 2:52(NIV)

52 And Jesus grew in wisdom and stature, and in favour with God and man

PRAYER FOCUS: Appreciate God for a new day. I bless you lord, because my baby shall, sit, talk, walk(mention others), at the right time. In Jesus name, Amen.

34

BE AN EXAMPLE

The faith of Timothy was traced to his mother and grand mother. He copied from his mum while the mom copied from her mom. In other words they were good role models. Do not forget that children practise easily what they see and they learn better by example. It can not be too early to model Christ to your baby. As you pray, as you sing, as you speak God's word, do not think that the baby is not noticing you. When he/she starts talking, you would understand that he/she has been learning. This is why it is necessary to create an atmosphere of love in the home. It is not enough to tell them what to do. Let them see you do it.

BIBLE READING AND MEDITATION
2 Timothy 1:5-I am reminded of your sincere faith, which first lived in your grandmother Lois

and in your mother Eunice and, I am persuaded, now lives in you also.

PRAYER FOCUS: Appreciate God for a new day. Father help me to be a good example to my child. Help me to point him/ her to you by my lifestyle. In Jesus name. Amen.

35

NO GENDER IS MORE IMPORTANT

With the mentality of some in our society that a male child is more important than the female, a lot of mothers end up getting so depressed when they discover that they are with a female child, especially if that is the 3rd, 4th or 5th where there is no male child. This could unconsciously reflect in our dealings with the innocent child. A friend told the story of how her mother, left her baby girl in the hospital after delivery because she wanted a boy after having 3 girls. Thank God for the father who discharged and cared for the baby girl. Today, that girl is a barrister, and the other sisters are doing so well with their husbands. Unfortunately, their mother died before most of them got married and the father is left to enjoy them.

BIBLE READING AND MEDITATION

Gal.3:28-There is neither Jew nor Gentile, neither slave nor free, nor is there male and female, for you are all one in Christ Jesus.

PRAYER FOCUS: Appreciate God for a new day. Lord I bless you for the sex of my baby. He/she is precious in your sight. He/she will fulfil purpose and destiny, no matter the gender. Thank you Lord. In Jesus name. Amen.

36

NO GENDER IS MORE IMPORTANT-2

The story above is a bit off normal as in most cases, it is the man that gets angry over the birth of a female child, forgetting that the Y chromosome which produces male children is usually from the man, not the woman. In any case, it is important to understand that before God there are no male or female, every one is equal. That is why He promised to release His Spirit upon sons and daughters alike. That is why, the daughters of Zelophedad were given a portion of their father's inheritance(Numbers 27:1-8). Mothers be excited over the baby you have got because many have been trusting God for decades just to have one. Celebrate your baby and love her/him (funny enough, some have so many boys and are trusting God for a girl). Trust God before you get pregnant for a desired sex, but give him praise for which ever sex He gives to you. Do not provoke God.

BIBLE READING AND MEDITATION

Gen.1:27-28-So God created mankind in his own image, in the image of God he created them; male and female he created them.

28 God blessed them and said to them, "Be fruitful and increase in number; fill the earth and subdue it. Rule over the fish in the sea and the birds in the sky and over every living creature that moves on the ground."

PRAYER FOCUS: Appreciate God for a new day. Father, thank you that my baby is special. (If your husband/ family is disappointed about the sex, commit them unto God's hands. That God will help them to appreciate God's gift.)

37

HELP BUILD SELF ESTEEM

A lot of children grow up with a perception that they are not loved. You have to start from now to show and express love to your baby. Smile at him/her, play with him/her, touch him/her to affirm love, cuddle, and always say, 'Ilove you". These would make your baby appreciate that you love him/her. Do not let your child, especially the females, hear the words, ' I love you" from others(especially boys) for the first time.

BIBLE READING AND MEDITATION
Titus 2:4-5
So that they may encourage the young women to love their husbands, to love their children, to be sensible, pure, workers at home, kind, being subject to their own husbands, so that the word of God will not be dishonored.

PRAYER FOCUS: Appreciate God for a new day. Lord, enable me to help my child to build good self esteem. May he /she grow up with emotional balance. May he/she always acknowledge that you love him/ her. In Jesus name. Amen

38

IN FAVOUR WITH MEN

An adage says "No one brings up a child alone, or a child does not belong to one person". It is practically impossible for you to be totally in charge of your baby always. Sometimes, even before the baby is 3 months, you might need the help of a nanny or baby seater to help take care of the baby due to your job etc.

.

Depend on God to give you people that would help you raise your children as if they were their own children, especially in this generation, when the women need to work. We encourage mothers to spend as much time as possible in commitment to raising their children. There must be times when you cannot help handing them over to someone's care: nanny, crèche etc. ,but you must endeavour to spend time with them at other times.

The decision to leave your baby under someone else's care could really be difficult to make and even so, one could be so anxious about what the said person could be doing to your baby. This is when you have to rely on God to cause men to favour your baby.

Learn to handover your baby to God every day. God in His mercies will not allow anyone do wrong to your children.

BIBLE READING AND MEDITATION

Ps 105: 14-15-He suffered no man to do them wrong: yea, he reproved kings for their sakes; Saying, Touch not mine anointed, and do my prophets no harm

Luke 2:,52(NIV)

52 And Jesus grew in wisdom and stature, and in favour with God and man

.

PRAYER FOCUS: Appreciate God for a new day. Lord, I ask that you grant my baby FAVOUR WITH MEN. No one will harm or hurt my baby.

Every caretaker will treat him/her as her own beloved child. In Jesus name. Amen.

39

DO NOT BE NEGLIGENT

God is able to keep your baby, but watch it, more than anything else, at this early stage and even in adulthood, your baby needs your attention. You do not have to be negligent. Do not leave the responsibility of raising your children to house helps, nannies and baby seaters. Never forget that a child will always pick up the habits and character of people they spend time with. Do not allow someone to determine the fate of your child, while you go after money. You might end up making the money, and losing your child, or having irresponsible children. Moreover, you have to be sensitive to the Holy Spirit and the signs God gives to you. If he prompts you to lay-off a nanny or baby seater, do so promptly. Delay of even a day might be too costly. You might lose your child. No job is more important than your baby. What would be your profit if you make the money and the baby is no more there to enjoy it. Many have resigned their jobs in order to take care of their babies; and they are happy today, reaping the rewards of good child upbringing. If your job is too demanding, that you have no time for your children, you might need to change it.

BIBLE READING AND MEDITATION
Titus 2:4-5 (KJV)

4 That they may teach the young women to be sober, to love their husbands, to love their children,

5 To be discreet, chaste, keepers at home, good, obedient to their own husbands, that the word of God be not blasphemed.

Prov 22:6Train up a child in the way he should go; even when he is old he will not depart from it.

PRAYER FOCUS: Appreciate God for a new day. God I thank you for the privilege to be a woman, wife and mother. Help me to be a good home keeper. I chose to take proper care of my family. Help me to be committed to my primary assignment. In Jesus name.Amen.

40

WHILE MEN SLEPT

The devil continually seeks whom to devour. Be a sensitive mother. A lot of babies who get initiated into the kingdom of darkness may have been free if their mothers were sensitive. According to people experienced in that area, initiation is a process which takes time and the baby usually reacts to it by falling ill, crying incessantly or unusually at night, being restless at night etc. That does not mean that whenever your baby cries at night, then he/ she is been initiated, but be sensitive. Instead of always explaining this off i.e. with your head and turning to the other side and continuing with your sleep, stand up and take some time to pray for your baby. Cover him/her with the blood of Jesus. Set his/her soul free from every demonic captivity.

BIBLE READING AND MEDITATION

I Peter 5:8-Be sober, be vigilant; because your adversary the devil, as a roaring lion, walketh about, seeking whom he may devour.

Matthew 13:25

But while everyone was sleeping, his enemy came and sowed weeds among the wheat, and went away. 26 When the wheat sprouted and formed heads, then the weeds also appeared.

PRAYER FOCUS: Appreciate God for a new day. Lord, I receive the grace to be vigilant and keep watch over my children, so that the enemy will not have grounds to speak reproachfully or rejoice over my children. In Jesus name. Amen

41

PALM TREES AND PILLARS

In a depraved generation like ours, with much juvenile delinquencies, God still promises that our young men will be like palm trees, and our daughters will be as pillars, POLISHED after the similitude of a palace. But who would do the polishing and who would tend the palm. It takes God and two P's to do this: patience and persistence. In other words, you have to keep doing your best, putting every effort continually, though sometimes stressful and you could be discouraged, to see that the future of your children are secured in God. Use the rod when necessary, but always let the child know why you are using it. Let them understand what they did wrongly, and correct in love. Teach them to apologize for mistakes and ask God for forgiveness when necessary.

BIBLE READING AND MEDITATION

Psalm144:12-(NIV) The sons in their youth will be like well-nurtured plants,

And our daughters will be like pillars carved to adorn a palace.

PRAYER FOCUS: Appreciate God for a new day. Lord, may my children bring honour to you and your kingdom. In Jesus name. Amen.

42

YOU CAN DO ALL THINGS

Make yourself available for God to use you even in "your condition" whether in pregnancy or while nursing your baby. The daughters God promised to use were not classified, whether they were to be single or married, pregnant or nursing mothers. Be strong. It is understandable, that sometimes, you might be too weak to do some things, but whenever you can, get committed. Do not lazy around and leave the ministry God has assigned to you. Plan your time properly. I once attended a program, and was thrilled, at how a pregnant lady was dancing, as she led the praise and worship session. I got to understand, that she was the choir leader. She was still committed to her ministry.

BIBLE READING AND MEDITATION
Phillipians 4:23-I can do all things, through Christ, who strengthens me.

PRAYER FOCUS: Appreciate God for a new day. I receive strength to do that which you expect of me always; doing the right thing at the right time. Thank you Lord. In Jesus name. Amen.

43

IT IS WELL

As a young mother, a lot of things might come up that bother you about your new baby; diaper rash, heat rash, atopic dermatitis, diarrhoea, fever, cough, catarrh; the list is endless. You need to cast your cares upon God, for He cares for you.

As we trust God for the best, sometimes, challenges come to put our faith to test. In times of challenges who do you look unto? When your child falls ill or a negative medical report is given, what do you do? Sit down and cry? No dear, there is still a God that reigns in the kingdoms of men. Hold on to Him.

The song writer wrote " I need thee, Lord, I need thee, every hour I need thee, oh bless me now my savior, I come to thee. Nursing a baby could be really demanding and strength draining. Each day, you need to ask God for fresh grace and strength.

BIBLE READINGAND MEDITATION

Isaiah 3:10(NIV)

Tell the righteous it will be well with them, for they will enjoy the fruit of their deeds.

Isaiah 8:18.Behold, I and the children whom the LORD hath given me are for signs and for wonders in Israel from the LORD of hosts, which dwelleth in mount Zion.

PRAYER FOCUS: Appreciate God for a new day. Lord I cast my cares upon you, because I know you care for me. I lay my burden down at your feet (mention what those cares are). Thank you Lord. In Jesus name. Amen.

44

TAKE IT BY FORCE

A woman of God once testified of how the baby in her womb had been confirmed dead. She was taken to the theatre to remove the dead baby. The devil told her she would die there. She did not keep silent but responded in a scream, that she shall not die. She confessed God's word and held on to it. Do you know that when she was operated on, in order to remove the baby, the baby screamed! It was as if it said "I am alive". The mother and baby came out alive and well. The violent takes it by force. Don't fold your hands and let the devil take that which belongs to you.

BIBLE READING AND MEDITATION
Matt 11:12-And from the days of John the Baptist until now the kingdom of heaven suffereth violence, and the violent take it by force.

PRAYER FOCUS: Appreciate God for a new day. Lord, I receive all that you have freely given to me in Christ Jesus. Satan take off your hold. In Jesus name. Amen.

45

YOU HAVE WHAT YOU SAY

Whoever says to the mountain be removed and cast to the sea, and shall not doubt in his heart, same shall have what he says(Mark 11:23). Let the redeemed of the Lord SAYso(Psalm 107:2). Women, I encourage you in this season of your life to begin to sow the seed of God's words (prophetic declarations) that you will reap its harvest in the future: harvest in the area of health, salvation, peace, progress of your child. Right there in the womb, in your arms as you carry/ cuddle your baby and all through life, continually declare God's word over that Child for scriptures says, God's word shall not return to him void, until it accomplishes the purpose of which it was sent(Isaiah 56:11) Declare over your child, you shall not die till you are a hundred years old(Isaiah 65:20). You shall be the head and not the tail, above only and never beneath(Deut. 28:13), you shall be an example to other believers(1Tim.

4:12), God will so satisfy you with the children's bread(healing) that you begin to live in health(Matt. 15:22-29). You shall be like a pillar, polished after the similitude of a palace (Psalm 144:12)

, no weapon formed or fashioned against you shall prosper (Isaiah 54:17). As you continually declare these words in faith, soon, you will see the manifestation.

BIBLE READING AND MEDITATION

Numbers 14:28- So tell them, 'As surely as I live, declares the LORD, I will do to you the very thing I heard you say:

PRAYER FOCUS: Appreciate God for a new day. Lord, according to your word in Psalm 127:4-5;Like arrows in the hands of a warrior are children born in one's youth.

5 Blessed is the man whose quiver is full of them, they will not be put to shame when they contend with their opponents in court. My children are arrows. I have victory in every situation concerning them. I am blessed, because of them. I shall not be ashamed in Jesus name. Amen.

46

IN PARTNERSHIP WITH GOD

Can you see from today's scripture that God is in need of a couple (you and your husband) that will help in raising a godly child? There was a time that God was angry and regretted that he created man, because his thought was evil continually(Genesis 6:5-6). He wanted a generation of people who would please him with their lifestyle. Unfortunately, a lot of children who have no regard for God are being raised.

I have always asked people, the armed robber, the cultist, the prostitute, the thief, the street fighter, if they were not born by mothers. If only they could meet God's need, of partnering with God to raise the children, they might not have ended that way. Mothers, see it as a privilege to partner with God in this ministry of raising godly children. May God be able to depend on you.

BIBLE READING AND MEDITATION

Malachi 2:15-And did not he make one? Yet had he the residue of the spirit. And wherefore one? That he might seek a godly seed. Therefore take heed to your spirit, and let none deal treacherously against the wife of his youth.

PRAYER FOCUS: Appreciate God for a new day. Lord, thank you for the privilege you have given to me, to partner with you in raising godly seed. Lord, may I not fail or disappoint you, in Jesus name. Amen.

47

IN PARTNERSHIP WITH GOD-2

The understanding that God is the one that called you into this ministry, should give you courage, knowing you are not alone in this business. God believed/trusted that Abraham would teach his children in His ways (Gen.18:19.). Can God trust you to raise up your children, pointing them to Jesus, the author and finisher of our faith? In moments when you become weary, why not you draw strength from the one who sent you on this errand. Like the Psalmist say, Lord, lead me to the rock, that is higher than I (Psalm 61:2). Remember, any business that God is involved in, never fails. Failure comes when you do it on your own, not involving God. Seek His help daily. The children are His heritage, He will not abandon them.

BIBLE READING AND MEDITATION

Psalm 127:3 -4"Children are a heritage from the Lord, offspring a reward from him. Like arrows in the hands of a warrior are children born in one's youth."

Deuteronomy 6:6-7 (NIV)

These commandments that I give you today are to be on your hearts. 7 Impress them on your children. Talk about them when you sit at home and when you walk along the road, when you lie down and when you get up.

PRAYER FOCUS: Appreciate God for a new day. Lord, I depend on you. Teach my children your ways. May they know you, the only true God, and Jesus Christ whom you have sent. May I ,and the children you have given me, be for signs and wonders in Israel.(Isaiah 8:18)

48

IT'S NOT TRUE

The greatest strategies of the devil are to steal, kill and destroy. He does this by speaking lies to people and if they believe and accept the lie, they are trapped in his web and they are doomed. Because the devil knows that the godly seed will break his head, he would do all things possible to destroy that seed. One of which is to speak a lot of lie to the mother who is the custodian of the child. Until a child gets to the age of accountability, most of what happens to the child, is determined by the custodian/parents. Because of this, the devil would come with lies: "your baby might develop congenital problems", "your child will die soon", "your baby might be infected with childhood diseases". You need to speak back woman. Do not be silent.

BIBLE READING AND MEDITATION

John 8:44-You belong to your father, the devil, and you want to carry out your father's desires. He was a murderer from the beginning, not holding to the truth, for there is no truth in him. When he lies, he speaks his native language, for he is a liar and the father of lies.

PRAYER FOCUS: Appreciate God for a new day. Lord, whatever the devil has spoken concerning my child are lies, and so, I decree that they shall not stand, neither shall they come to pass. In Jesus name. Amen.

49

IT'S NOT TRUE-2

A man of God said, while the wife was pregnant, he said : "what if the child has a palate problem (cleft palate)". The devil must have been the one that whispered that to his mind, and he carelessly spoke it out. Sure enough, the devil worked on what he said, and the child was actually born with a palate problem. Whenever the devil speaks to you, learn to counter it with God's word. That is why you are encouraged to have a store of God's word in your heart by daily meditation. When the devil then speaks, as he always will, you get the appropriate reply and speak it back to him. He sure will flee immediately.

In a world, where so many lives have been cut short due to childhood diseases, accident, one form of misfortune or the other, God's word still remains true. The mother could sometimes be filled with fear of what could become of her baby. Instead of allowing the devil to fill your heart with thoughts of fear, and thereby having ground to bring such to pass, speak God's word.

BIBLE READING AND MEDITATION
Lamentations 3:37 (K J V)

Who is he that saith, and it cometh to pass, when the Lord commandeth it not?

PRAYER FOCUS: Appreciate God for a new day. Father, your words are yea and amen. I believe your word concerning my child. I cancel every negative statement that I, or anyone else has made concerning my child. They shall not stand, neither shall they come to pass, in Jesus name. Amen.

50

SHE BRINGETH HER FOOD FROM AFAR.

One of the virtues of the virtuous woman is her ability to provide food for the home from "Afar". To me, it speaks of her ability to get or source for the food where it is cheapest (Still putting transportation cost in mind and stress of going there into consideration). As a nursing mother, or a pregnant woman, feeding is a major area of concern for the mother and baby. This could cost a lot of money; since the mother has to be on fruits, milk (a pregnant woman should take a glass of milk daily) etc. to have a healthy baby. Wisdom demands that you reduce cost as much as possible. Get what you need from places where they are less expensive. Why would you buy a tin of milk from a nearby shop for N750, when you know you can get it at N600 else where (without putting in much stress and money to go there). If it is possible, why not you get four at a time, instead of going to this "far" place every week. You can also plan to buy everything you need when you go for shopping, instead of buying things in bits. If it will not be too much for you, why not you prepare your baby's pap yourself. You can save cost and you will be sure that your baby is eating hygienically prepared pap. Note also that the expensive and classy baby food are not 'necessarily' the best. If you cannot afford them, do not feel bad. You can get cheaper substitutes which would do the same job.

BIBLE READING AND MEDITATION
Prov.31:14-She is like the ships of the merchant; she brings her food from afar.

PRAYER FOCUS: Appreciate God for a new day. Father God, I receive wisdom for prudence. In Jesus name. Amen.

51

EAT AND DRINK, FOR THE JOURNEY IS FAR

God's word spoken and applied at the right time guarantees victory.(Jn 1:3).Without the word, nothing is created. You have to declare God's words to ensure a successful pregnancy. You need God's word for safe delivery, you need God's word for a healthy baby, you need God's word all the way. But do you have to wait for challenges to come or the time you need the word before you get the word? Jesus was able to overcome the devil because He knew the word before the temptation came. All he needed to do was to apply the word. Women, continually give yourself to the study of God's word so you can speak the right word in due season. A lot of people make the mistake of looking for the right scripture to use, when the devil is already on their case. Even if they get the word then, they speak it out of fear, instead of faith, and end up in defeat. That will not be your case in Jesus name, Amen.

BIBLE READING AND MEDITATION

1 Kings 19:7-The angel of the LORD came back a second time and touched him and said, "Get up and eat, for the journey is too much for you."

PRAYER FOCUS: Appreciate God for a new day. Lord, I receive the grace to study, to show myself approved, a workman that does not need to be ashamed, rightly dividing the word of truth.(2 Tim. 2:15)

52

PRAY AHEAD

Elijah was told in a dream; eat and drink for the journey is far. Jesus told Peter—the devil has planned to sift you like wheat, but I have prayed for you. Our prayer goes a long way to settle things in the future when made early. A prayerful parent clears the way and makes life "easier" for the child. There are some people who fight battles in life and face lots of obstacles as a result of what their ancestors might have done. But those who are offspring of godly/prayerful parents enjoy peace. That is because, their prayerful parents clear the spiritual atmosphere for their children. They break known or unknown curses, destroy evil altars, break negative covenants, etc. Make use of every opportunity to sow seeds of prayer into the future of your child. While breast feeding, while bathing him or her, while rocking the child etc. instead of singing some meaningless songs to keep the baby calm, compose and sing songs of prayers;

pray about everything and every phase of life;health, academics, marriage, ministry. Prophesy into the future of the child.

BIBLE READING AND MEDITATION
1King 19:7

The angel of the LORD came back a second time and touched him and said, "Get up and eat, for the journey is too much for you."

Matt.26:41-"Watch and pray so that you will not fall into temptation. The spirit is willing, but the flesh is weak."

PRAYER FOCUS: Appreciate God for a new day. Lord, I receive grace to be committed to praying for my children. I shall sow the seeds of prayer into their destiny, and in due season, I shall reap. In Jesus name. Amen.

53

PRAY AHEAD-2.

If care and adequate spiritual/prayerful steps are not taken, there is every tendency for negative traits in you or your parents to be repeated in your children. In Gen 49:5-7, Jacob, cursed the anger of Levi, which made him to kill all the men in a city. In Ex 2:1-2, we understand that Moses is from the house of Levi, and same anger, prevented him from entering into the promised land. Also, Sarah, Abram's wife was barren(Gen. 16:1). Likewise, Rebecca, the daughter in law, (Gen 25:21), likewise Rachael, the daughter in law to Isaac (Gen 30:1). Do you also know, that in Gen 12:13, Abram told Sarah to claim to be his sister for fear that they might kill him for her sake?In Gen. 26:7; Isaac also claimed that Rebecca was his sister for fear that he might be killed. Dear, if you refuse to take your stand in prayer, negative traits in your lineage are bound to be repeated in your children. You need to investigate and be sensitive to what those traits are, and pray against their manifestation in the life of your children.

BIBLE READING AND MEDITATION
Jeremiah 31:29-30 (NIV)

29 "In those days people will no longer say, 'The parents have eaten sour grapes,

and the children's teeth are set on edge.'
30 Instead, everyone will die for their own sin; whoever eats sour grapes their own teeth will be set on edge.

PRAYER FOCUS: Appreciate God for a new day. Father, I decree, that my child/ children shall not inherit any negative trait or habit from me or his/her ancestors(paternal or maternal). He/she is delivered from every curse, operating in his/ her family (paternal/ maternal), by the blood of Jesus. In Jesus name. Amen.

54

A GODLY SEED

The reason God brought the man and woman together is that they might raise a godly seed(Mal. 2:15). A seed that will fulfill God's purpose and destiny.A seed that will bring glory to God. A seed that will depopulate hell and populate God's kingdom. It is the responsibility of the parents to raise this seed. Parenthood is work; it is hard work. It does not end in providing the needs of food/shelter, school fees etc. You have to ensure that the child is brought up in God's ways. As the baby grows, note that the "rod" must be applied when necessary, prayers must be made to ensure God's reign in the life of the child and the right lifestyle must be modeled to the child.

BIBLE READING AND MEDITATION
Prov. 22:6 Train up a child in the way he should go, and when he is old, he will not depart from it.

Deuteronomy 6:7-9 (NIV)

7- Impress them on your children. Talk about them when you sit at home and when you walk along the road, when you lie down and when you get up. 8 Tie them as symbols on your hands and bind them on your foreheads. 9 Write them on the doorframes of your houses and on your gates.

PRAYER FOCUS: Appreciate God for a new day. Lord God, I receive the grace to raise children that will honour and serve you all the days of their life. In Jesus name. Amen.

55

POWER IN THE BLOOD

The blood which Jesus shed on the cross of Calvary remains one of the most powerful weapons of our warfare. Today's scripture speaks of the victory over the dragon who wanted to destroy the man child born by the woman. By the blood of Jesus, be rest assured that you will always triumph. But you have to be sure that you have the right to war with the blood; if you have claims to use it. I mean, if you are born-again. If not, even if you plead an ocean full of the blood, the enemy will still defeat you. Surrender your life to Christ today.

BIBLE READING AND MEDITATION

Rev.12:11" and they overcame him by the blood of the lamb and by the word of their testimony.

PRAYER FOCUS: Appreciate God for a new day. (If you have not received Jesus as your Lord and personal saviour, here is another opportunity to do so. Say this prayer : Father, I thank you for sending your son Jesus, to die for my sins. Lord Jesus, I receive you today as my Lord and personal saviour. Father, forgive me all my sins. Cleanse me with the blood of Jesus. Cancel my name from the book of death, and write it in the book of life. Satan, I reject you and your works. In Jesus name. Amen. Father I thank you for the victory I have, by the blood of Jesus. I cover my life and my child/children with the blood of Jesus. We are victorious. In Jesus name. Amen.

56

SOME CHALLENGES NURSING MOTHERS FACE, AND TIPS ON HOW TO HANDLE THEM.

1. **NOT GETTING ENOUGH SLEEP/REST-** This is often the case, due to the fact that you always have to breastfeed the baby, or attend to him/her when crying, either night or day. To handle this, try to sleep while the baby sleeps. Let someone care for the baby, while you get some much needed rest. It would also be necessary to set some rules with respect to visitors. Like, time for visit and how long they stay. You could also insist that no one should wake you up if a visitor comes while you are sleeping. It would also be necessary to plan a schedule with your spouse: who takes care of the baby at night, etc. Also, do not be too rigid about meeting expectations. If you are too tired to prepare the regular meal for the family, please, appeal to them

to make do with an alternative. If you are too tired to arrange items in the house, excuse yourself and rest, instead of breaking down. The laundering must not be done NOW. G ive yourself a break.

2. **MOOD SWING**-It is normal for a nursing mother to have mood swings; excited in a moment about the new baby, and a short while later, feeling bad over the stress involved in taking care of the baby, and how you are restricted because of the baby. To handle that, get emotional support from your husband. Get hugs and kisses as you need them. Learn to do something you enjoy daily; take some time out for a walk; have outdoor fun time with the family; talk to someone that cares and always know that it is only for a season. Also acknowledge that it is a privilege to mother a child.

3. **FEELINGS OF EXHAUSTION**: Caring for the newborn requires energy. Take care of yourself- get healthy diet, drink plenty of

water, get fresh air. Get help from relatives, friends, nanny e.t.c

4. **ILL FEELINGS TOWARDS YOUR HUSBAND**: Sometimes, some women develop ill feelings towards their husbands, out of the stress of nursing a baby. You might be expecting your husband to help in so many ways, while he might be carried away with his job and how to provide for the home. To handle this; excuse your spouse, remember the ways he has helped and tell yourself he is doing his best. Also, talk things over with him. Let him know your expectations. Both of you should come to understanding of what each of you is expected to do per time. Learn to spend time together to nurture your relationship. Always appreciate him. No matter how much time and commitment your baby requires, make out time to attend to your husband, knowing that the baby will someday grow-up and leave the house for you and your husband.... if Christ tarries. Attend to his emotional needs. Love him.

5. **YOUR SHAPE IRRITATES YOU**. The stretch marks, extra fat deposits, large breasts,e.t.c. might weigh you down. Some feel that their husband wouldn't like them anymore. To handle that, you can share your concern with your husband. He likely will re-assure you of his love. Do not crash diet and get involved in intensive exercise to lose the weight within a short while. You would gradually lose the weight, just as it did not take you just a day to gain it. Also, be encouraged that added fat deposit and a bigger breast are actually needed in helping you to nurse your baby and have enough energy for coping with the challenges of having a new baby. Let the joy of motherhood, overwhelm you.

6. **BREASTFEEDING**: It could sometime be frustrating especially with getting the timing and positioning. Give yourself time to learn, may be about a month, as it gets easier with time. Get counsel from another mom who has nursed children. She could watch to see if you are doing it right.

BENEFITS OF BREAST FEEDING

Many medical experts strongly recommend breastfeeding exclusively (no formula, juice, or water) for 6 months. And breastfeeding for a year at least with other foods which should be started at 6 months of age, such as vegetables, grains, fruits, proteins. According to the American Academy of Pediatrics and the American College of Obstetricians and Gynecologists, the benefits of breastfeeding are as follows:

THE BENEFITS OF BREASTFEEDING FOR THE BABY

1. Breast milk provides the ideal nutrition for infants. It has a nearly perfect combination of everything your baby needs to grow.

2 It is provided in a form more easily digested by the baby compared to infant formula.

3 Breast milk contains antibodies that help your baby fight off viruses and bacteria and other diseases.

4 Some studies show that breastfeeding is linked to higher Intelligence Quotient scores in later childhood.

5 The closeness and physical contact between the mother and child during breastfeeding, helps with bonding and makes the baby feel secure.

6 Breastfed infants are more likely to gain the right amount of weight as they grow rather than become overweight children.

7 Breastfeeding plays a role in the prevention of sudden infant death syndrome (SIDS).

BENEFITS OF BREASTFEEDING FOR THE MOTHER

1. Breastfeeding burns extra calories, so it can help you lose pregnancy weight faster.

2. It releases the hormone oxytocin, which helps your uterus return to its pre-pregnancy size and may reduce uterine bleeding after birth.
3. Breastfeeding also lowers your risk of breast and ovarian cancer.
4. Breastfeeding may also lower your risk of osteoporosis.
5. Breast feeding is cost effective and saves time. This is because you do not have to buy and measure formula, warm bottles or sterilize nipples . It also gives you regular time to relax quietly with your newborn.

ABOUT THE AUTHOR

Dr Mrs. Ufuooma Nwachukwu Onwuka , an optometrist by profession has a strong youth and relationship-oriented ministry. She is the president of True Love Club of Nigeria and the host of an annual Valentine Youth Programme (TRUE LOVE CONFERENCE). She is the author of the Celebrated Woman and The Path of Righteousness. She is happily married to Pastor Kingsley Onwuka and they are blessed with four children. She resides in Enugu, Nigeria.

www.ingramcontent.com/pod-product-compliance
Lightning Source LLC
Chambersburg PA
CBHW020320290526

45785CB00007B/2852